This book is dedicated to those affected by the sudden loss of an important person.
Please, if you feel any thoughts of hurting yourself, call 988 or text life to 741741.
You are wanted.

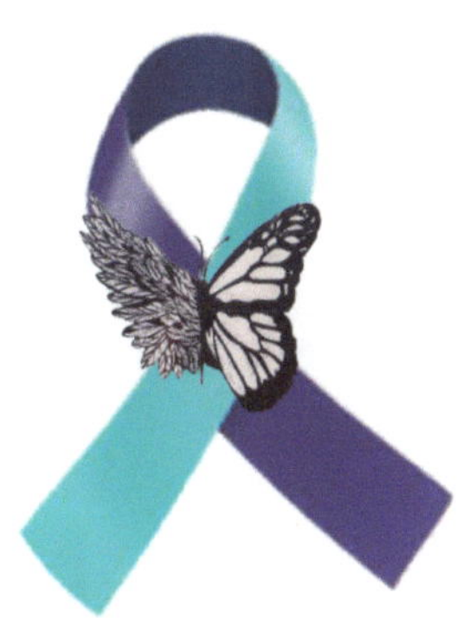

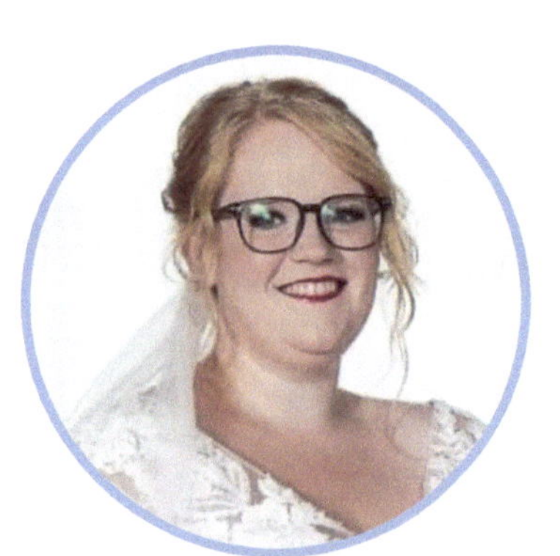

About the author: Brittany is a children's book writer and special education teacher in Minnesota. Her and her husband made it their goal to be able to help other kids deal with loss after the sudden loss of his dad.

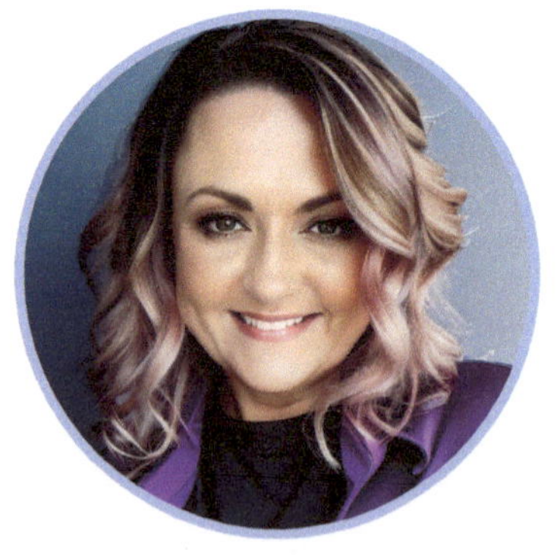

About the illustrator: Cassie is a wife, mother, and local artist in Utah. She has been drawing since she was little and loves to capture the world from a child's eye. She finds hope and inspiration as she brings visions to life.

Why are you sleeping?
I still need you here.

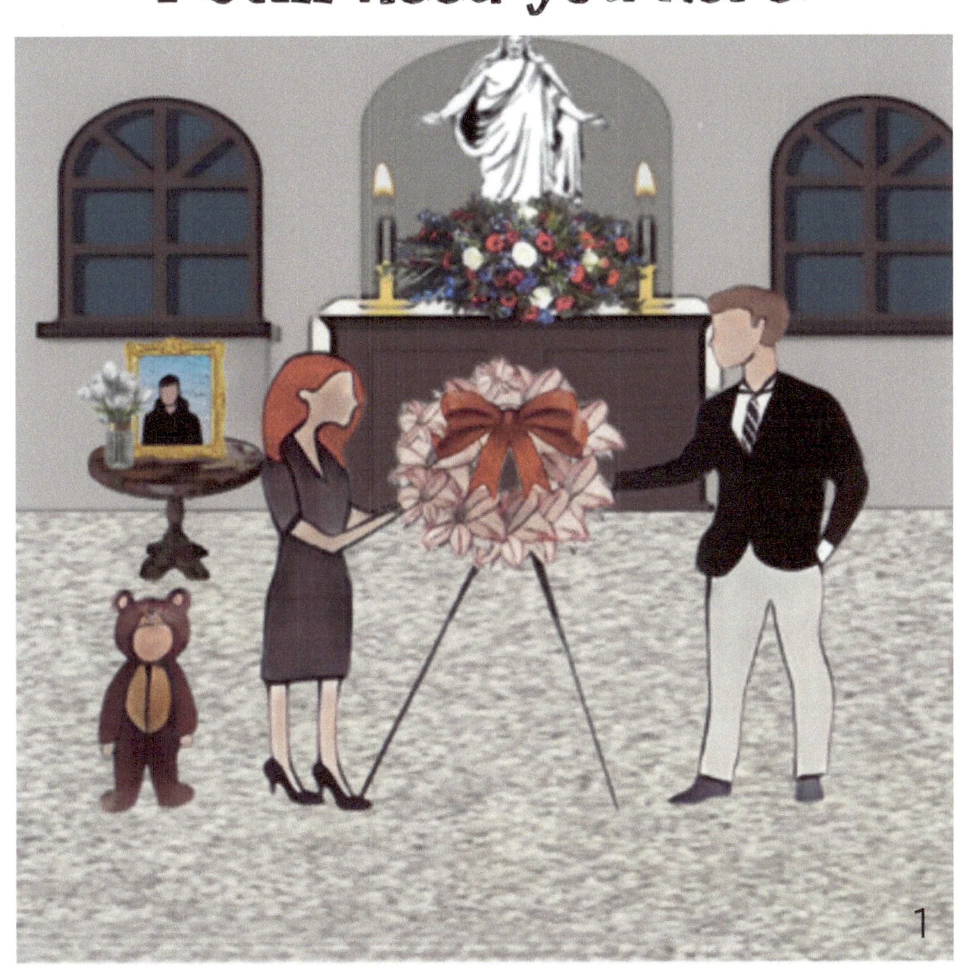

They say you are gone,
but I know you'll
appear.

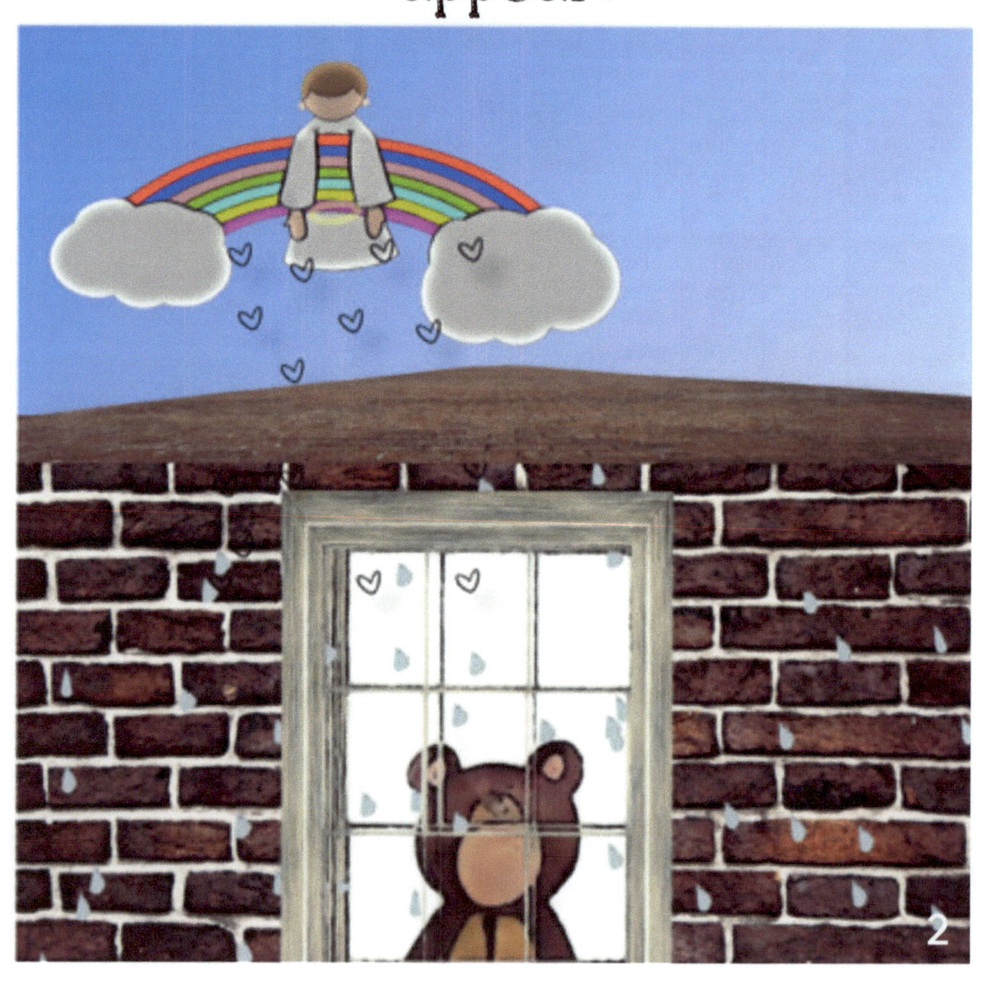

So why do they say
you won't come
back ever?

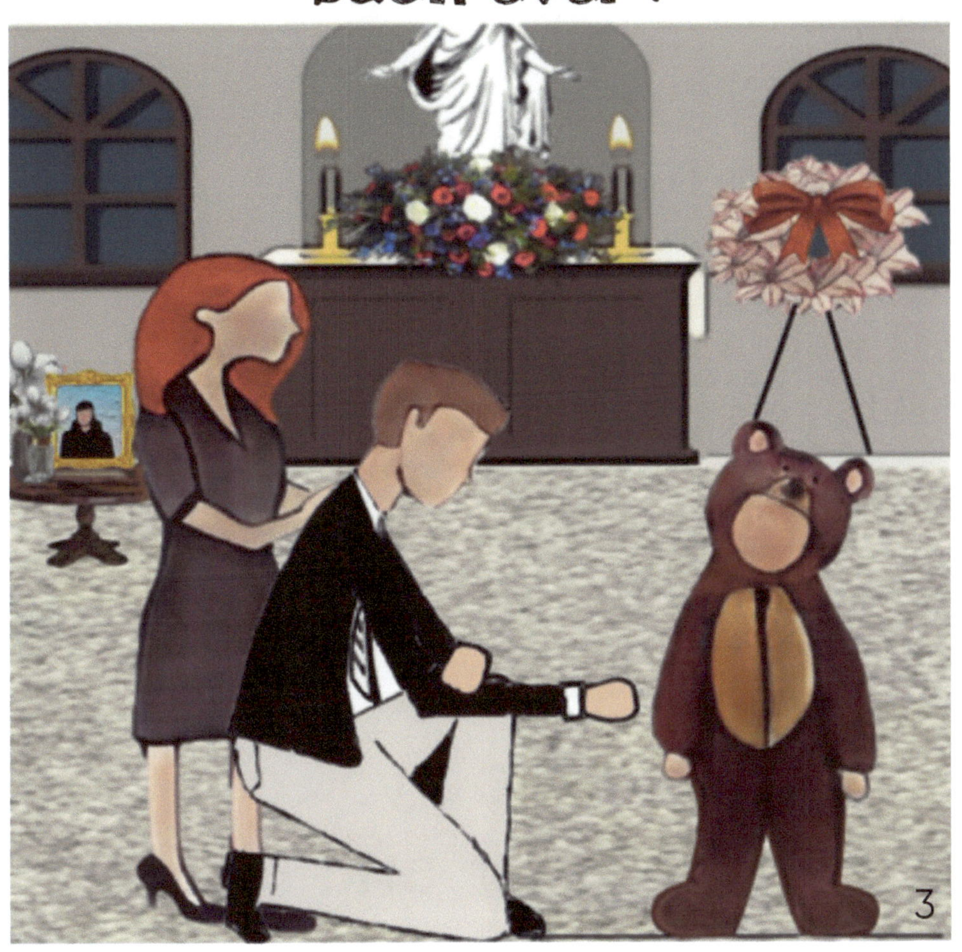

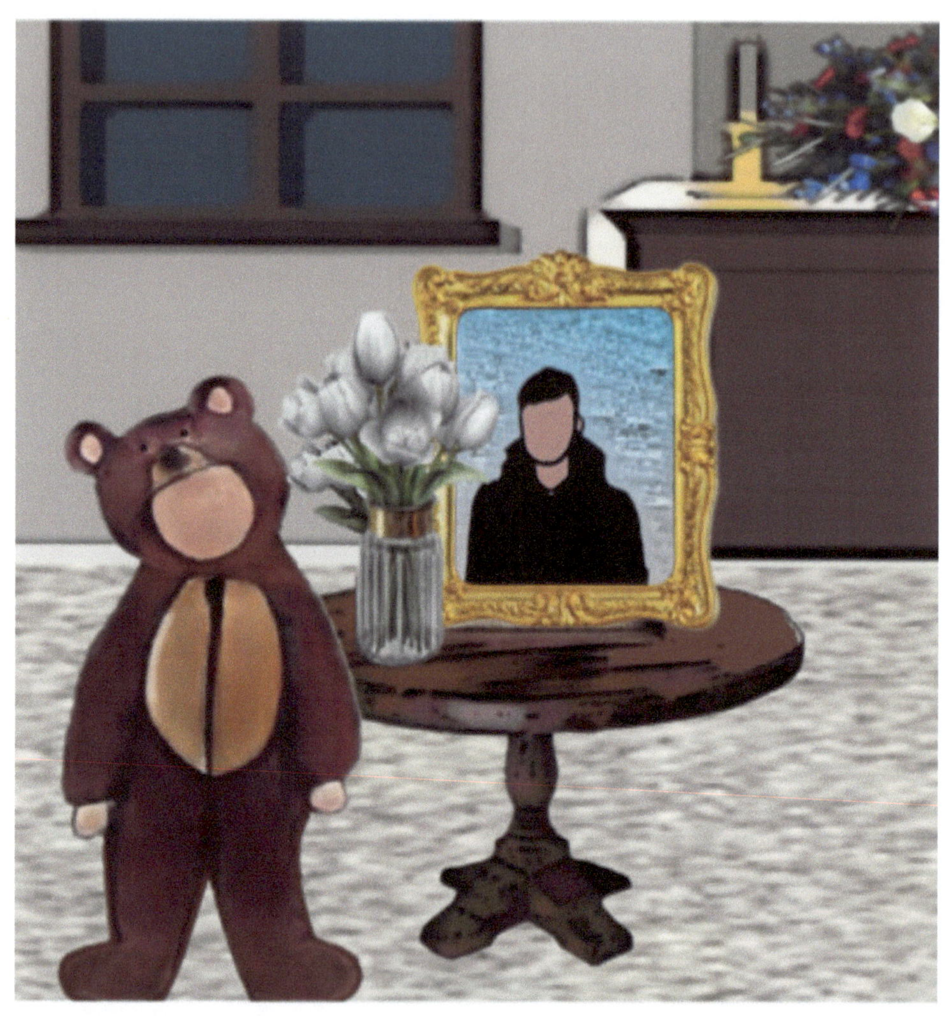

You said that you'd love
me forever and ever..

Why are you
sleeping?
I need you to play.

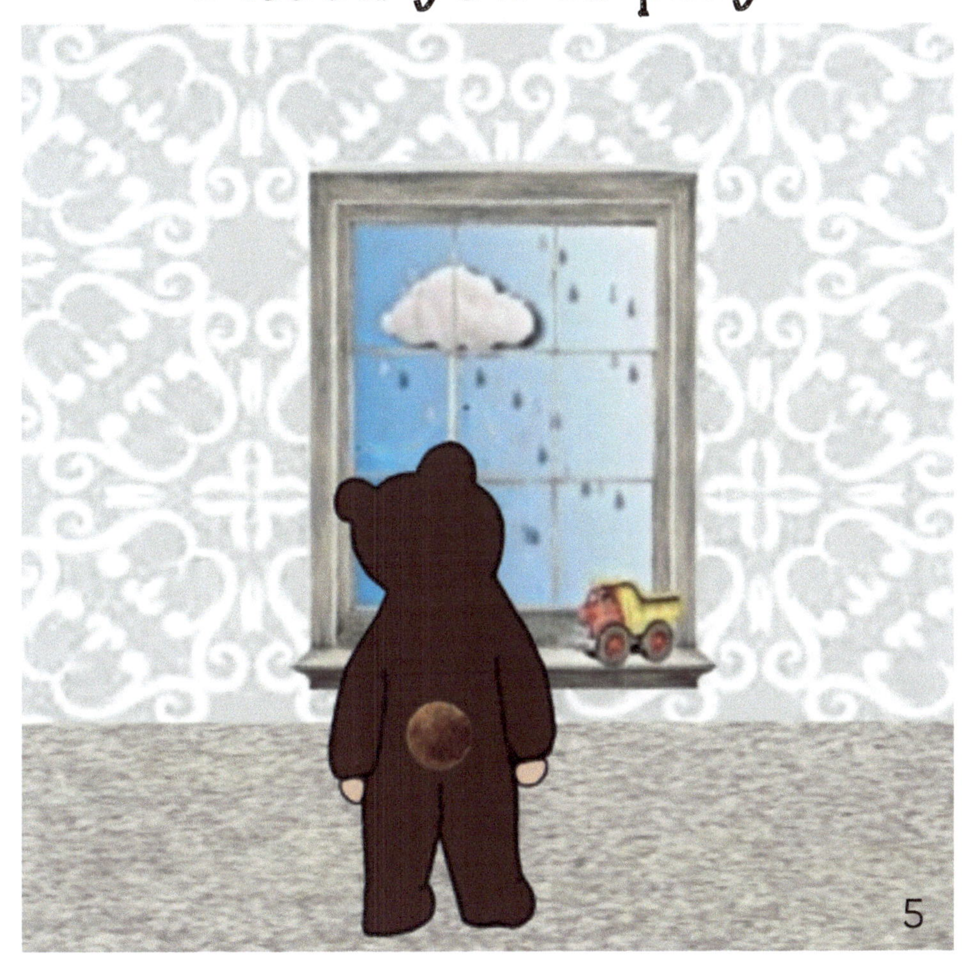

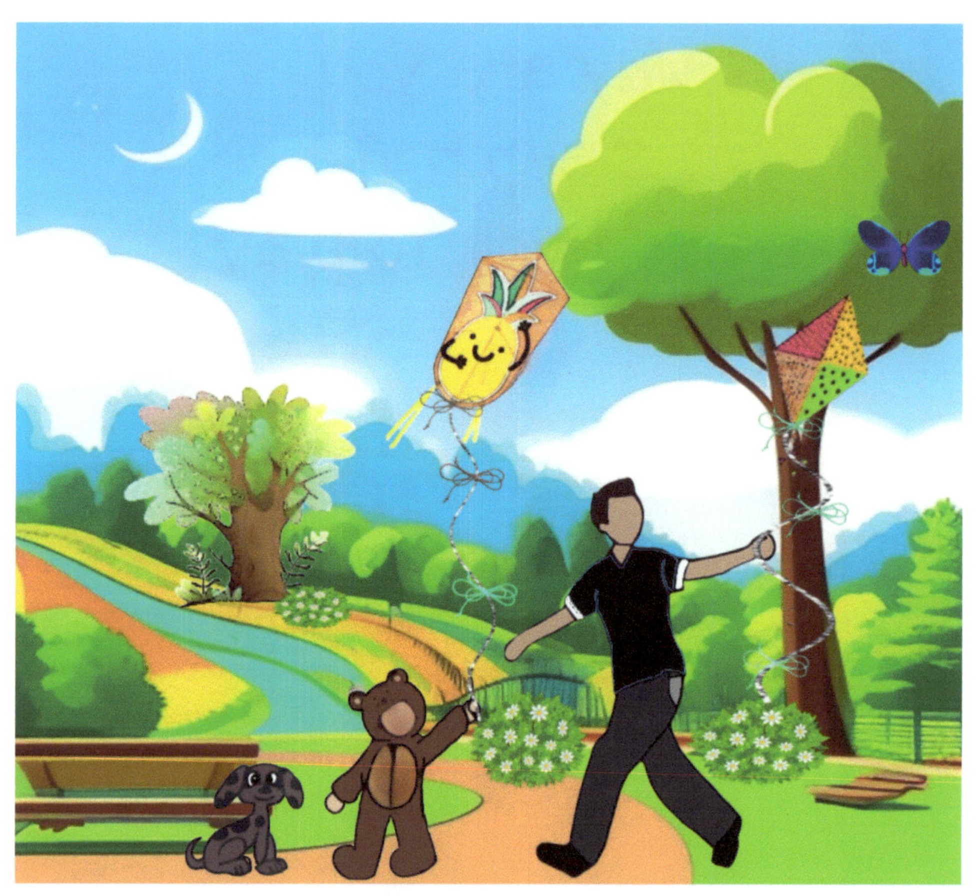

Come catch me and laugh,
while I run, acting tough. We
will roll in the grass. as the
moon comes up!

Why are you
sleeping? I need
your bear hugs.

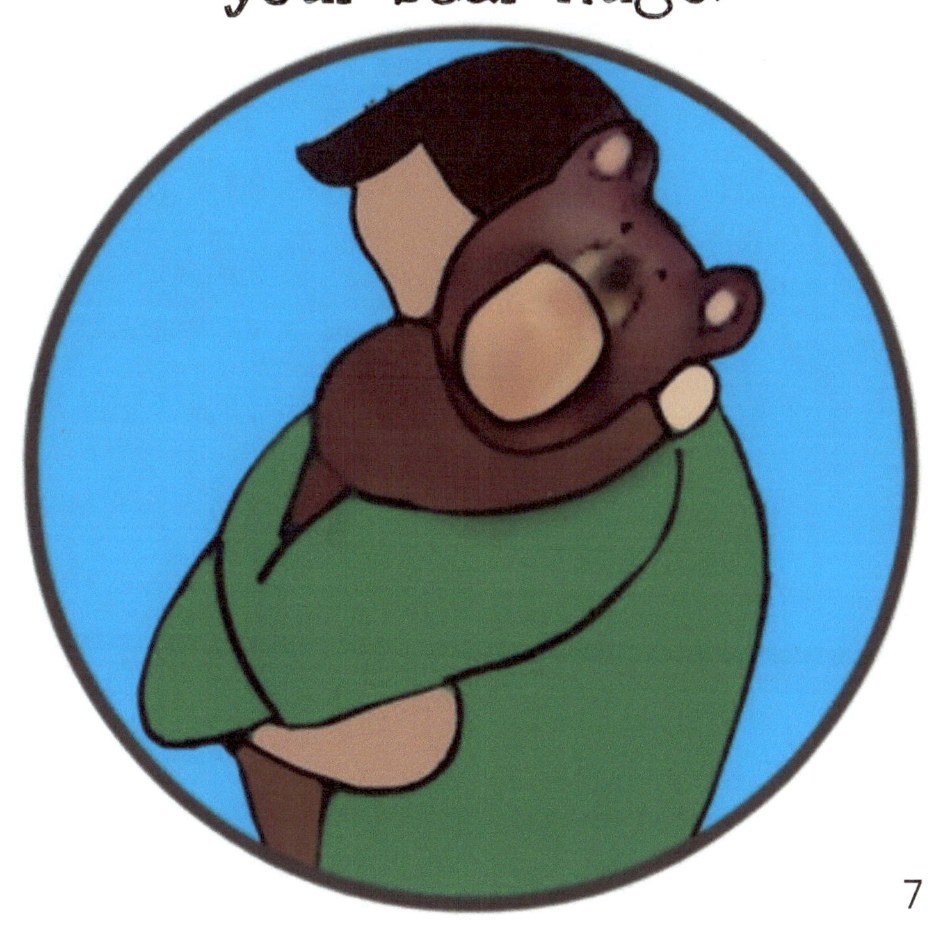

7

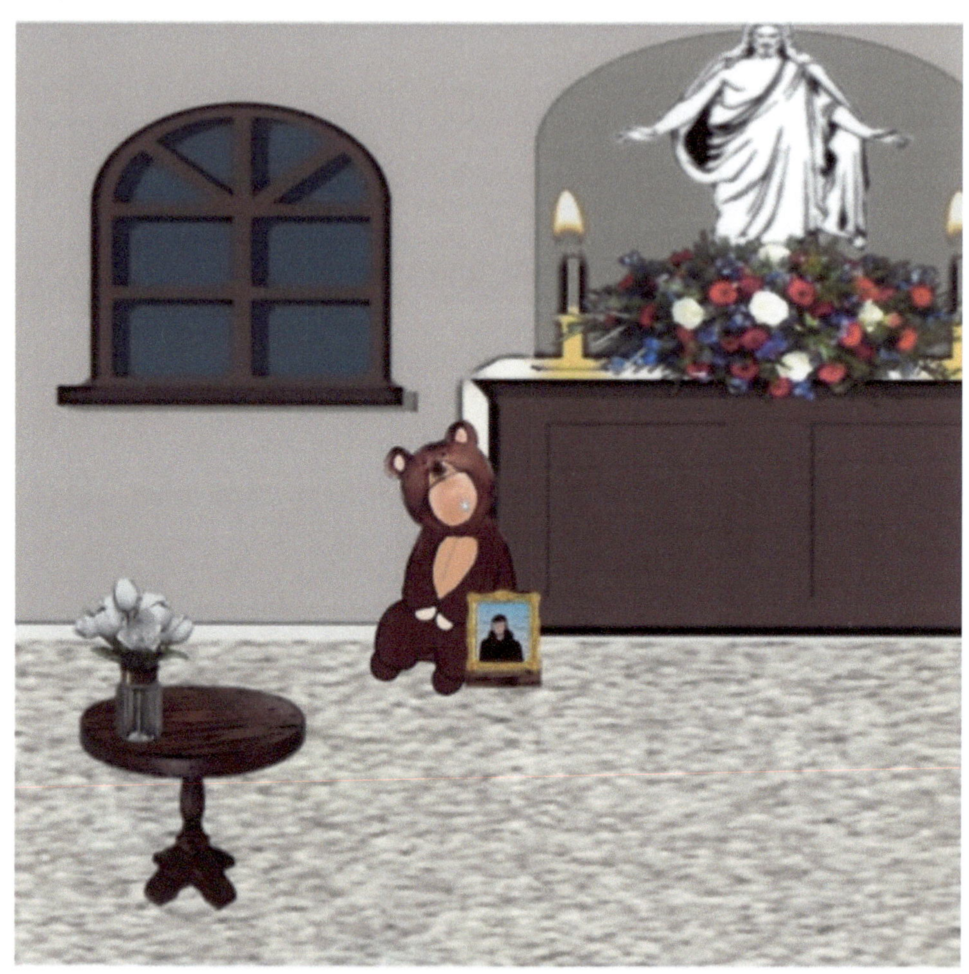

When I'm tired and
sleepy, when I'm
down or in love. 8

I need you to tell me it will
be alright. I need you to
come here and hold me tight.

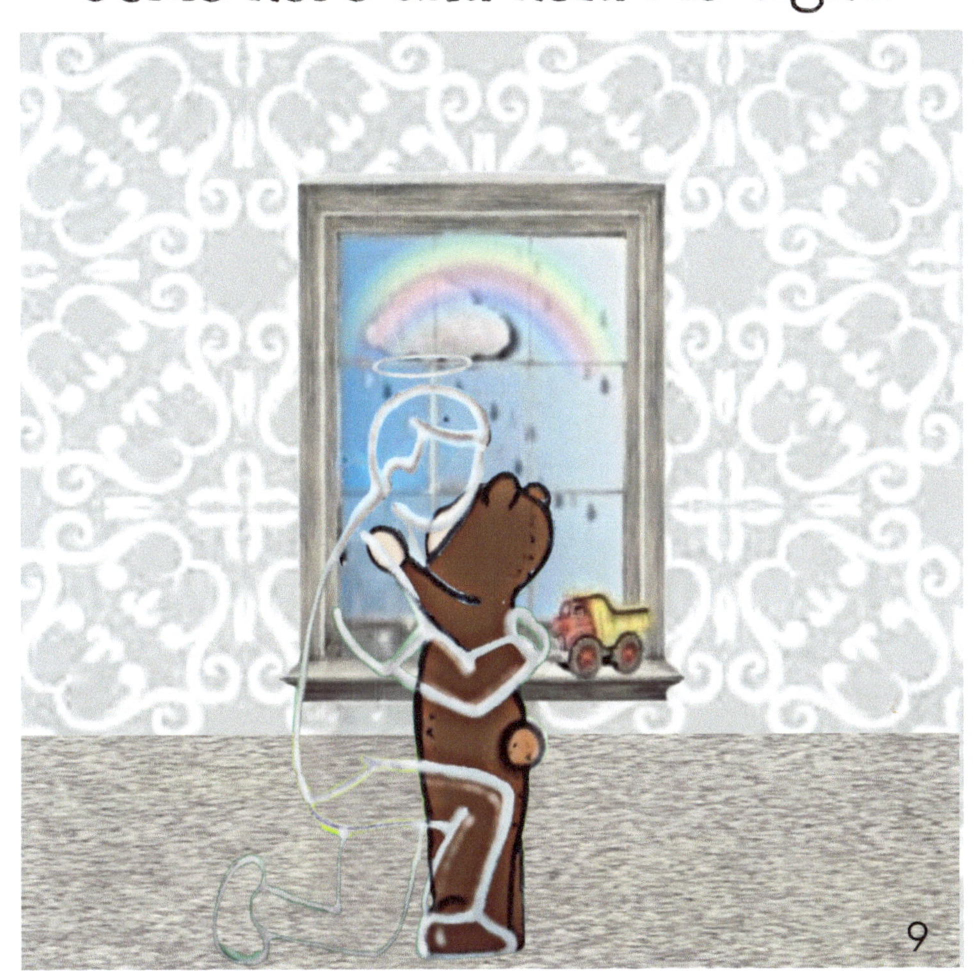

I need you to wake up, I need you
with me. You're supposed to be
here. So why are you sleeping?

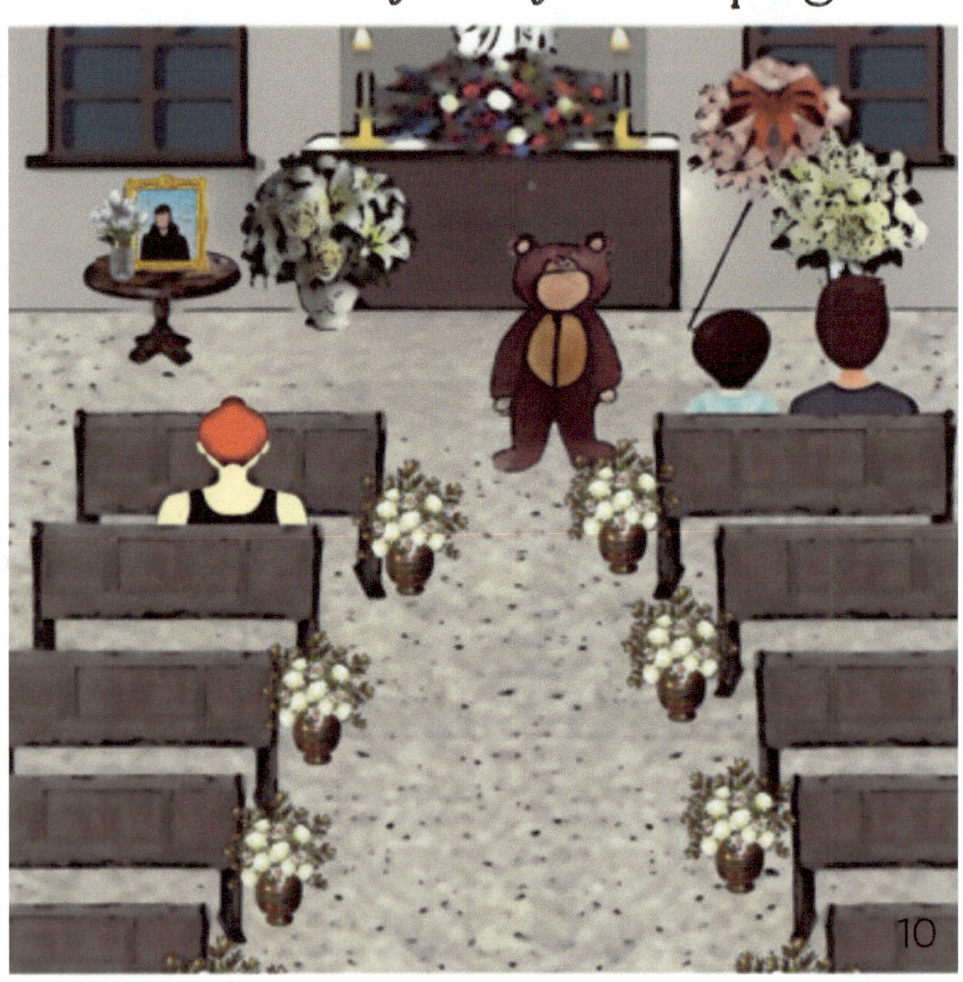

Why are you sleeping?
The sun is out now.

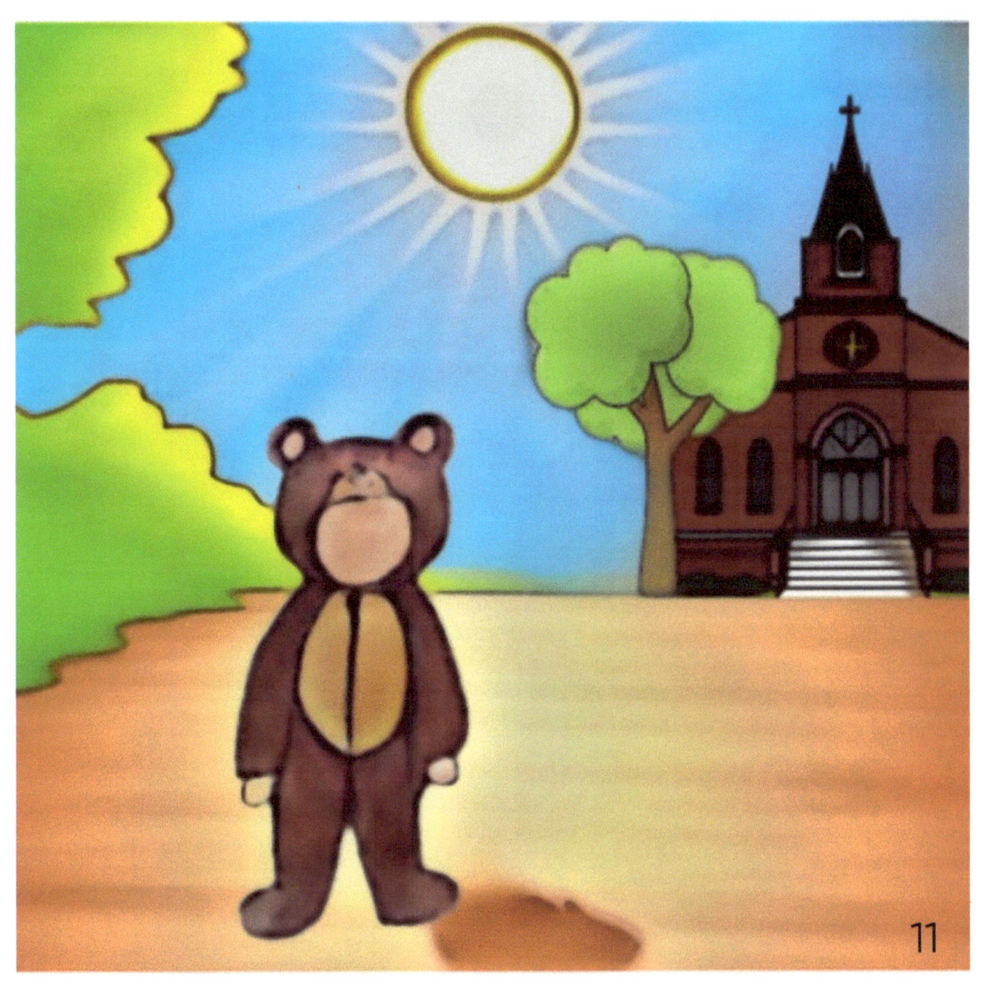

The world is warming, it's your
favorite time of year.

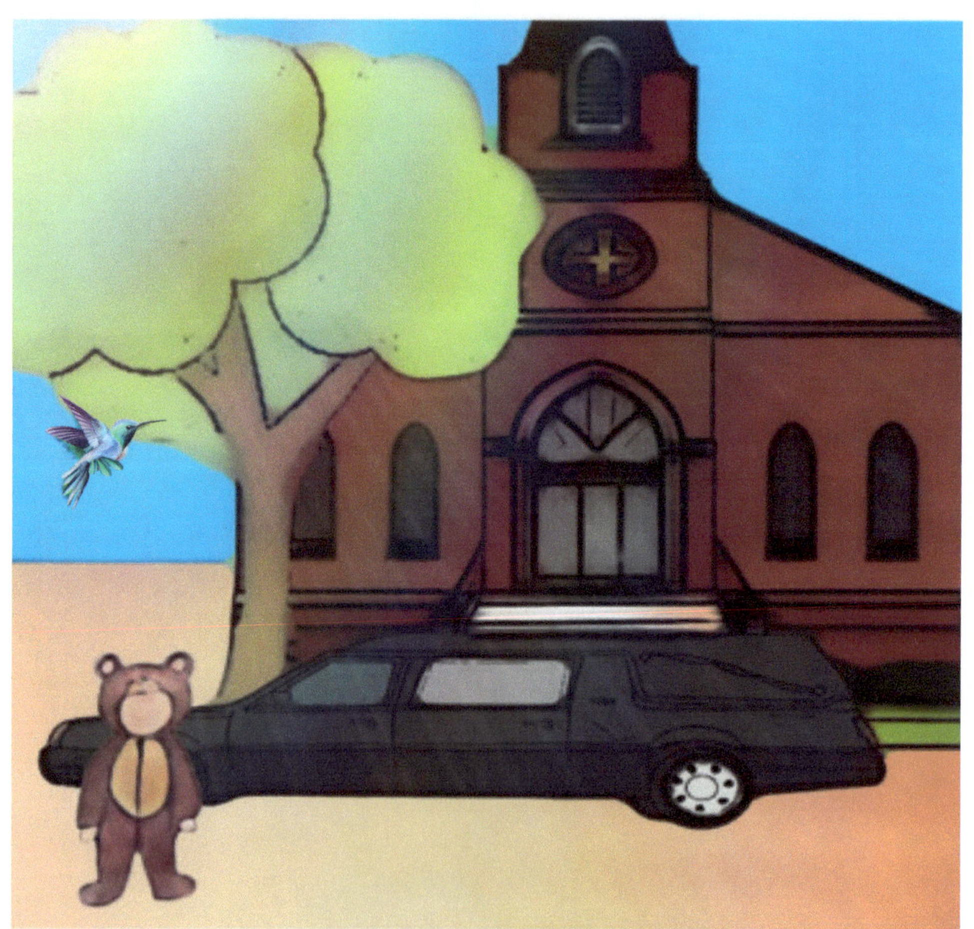

Why are you sleeping?
You should be here.

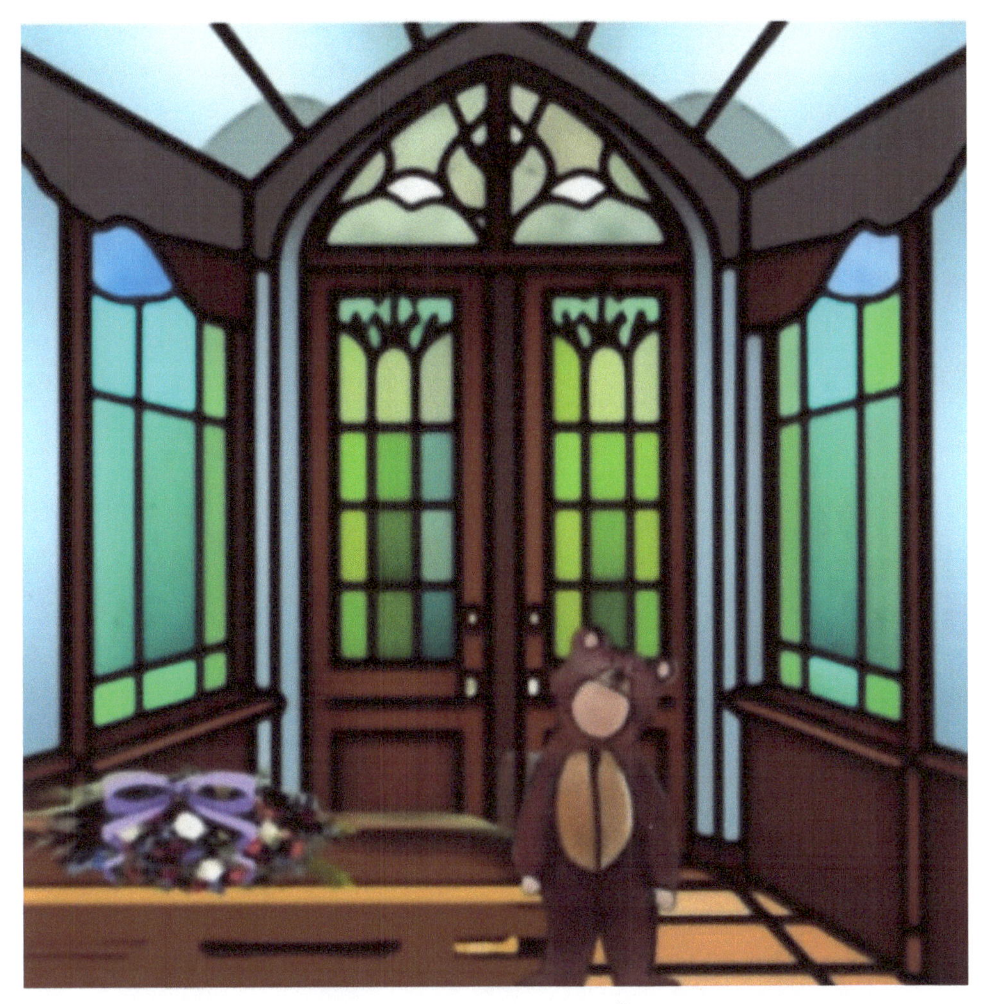

Why are you sleeping
in that big wooden bed?

Everyone is
crying and bowing
their heads.

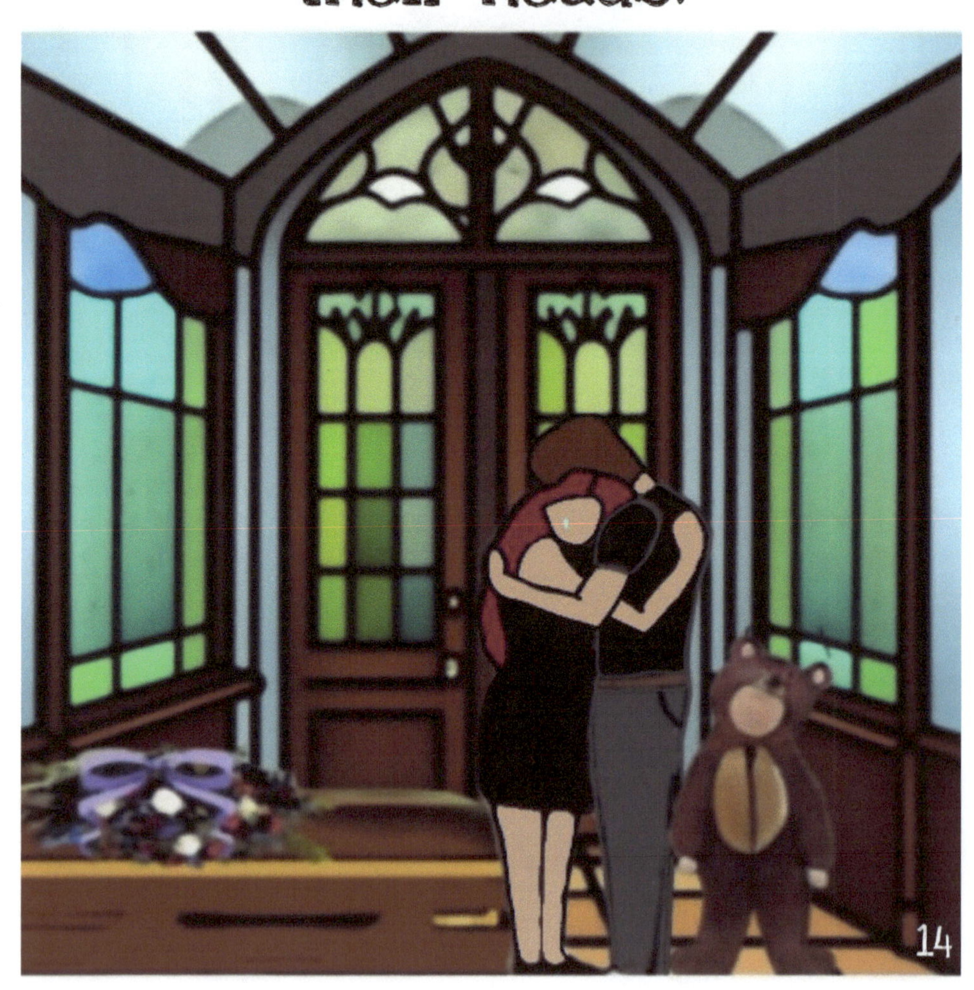

Why are you sleeping?
Why won't you wake?

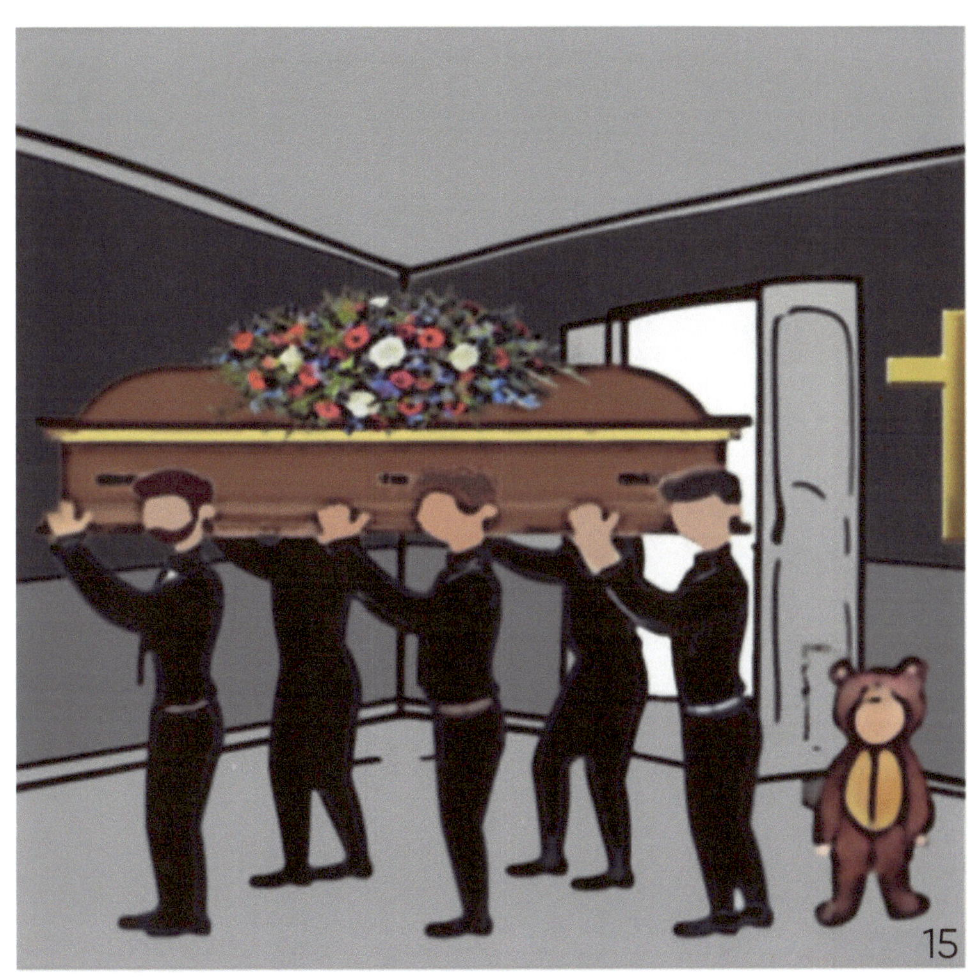

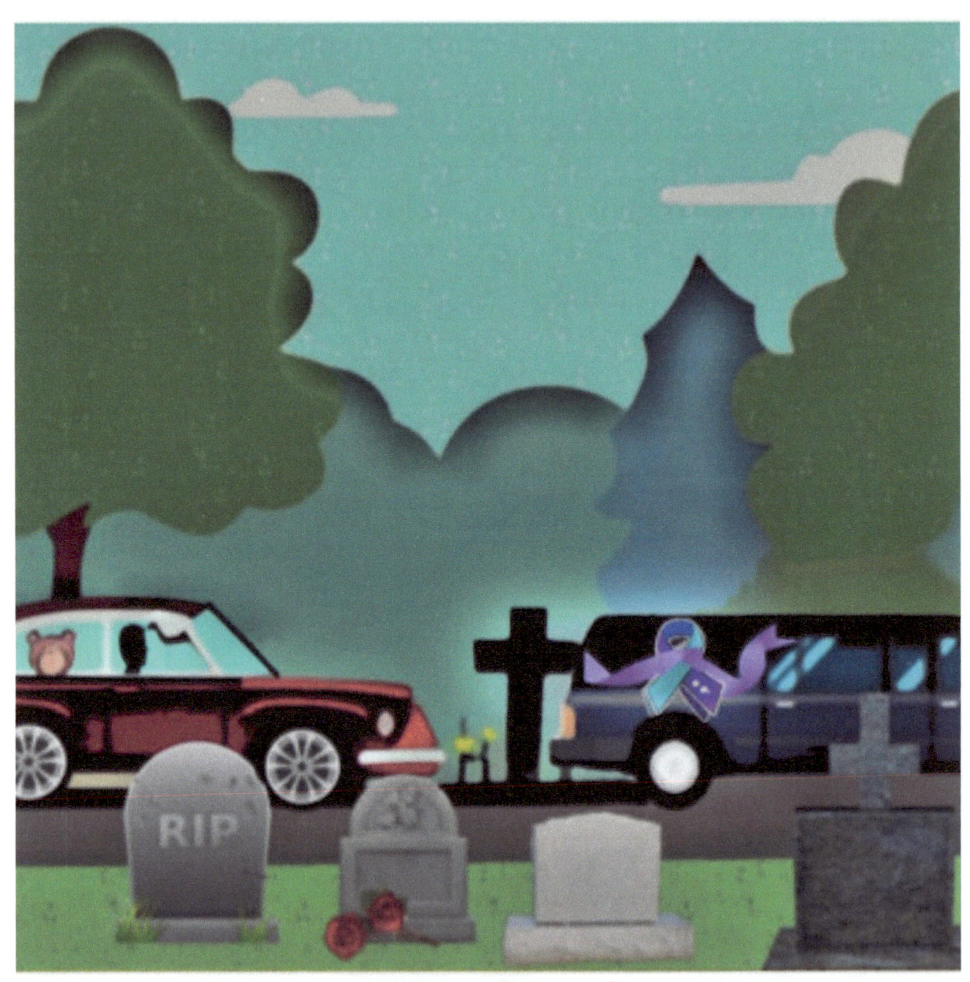

They say that you
did this, but that
can't be your fate.

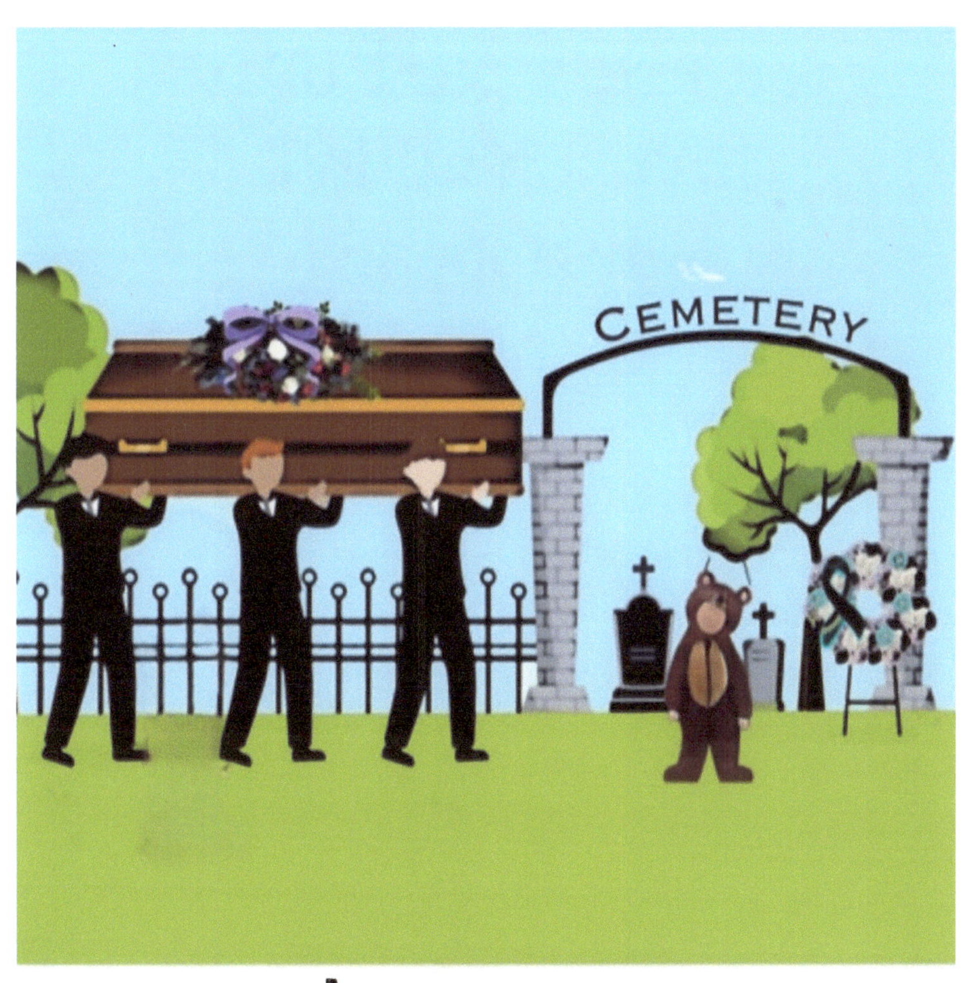

Why are you
sleeping?
We needed you here. 17

You are a part of us
that shouldn't
disappear.

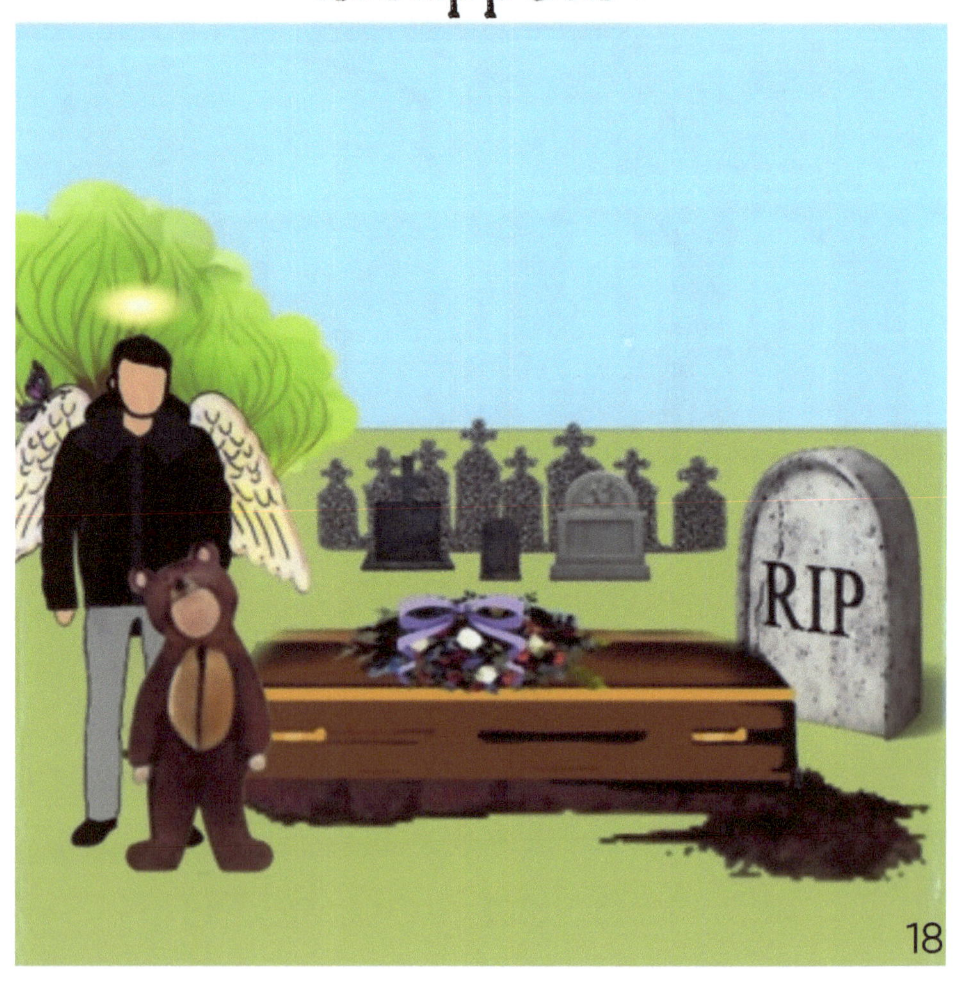

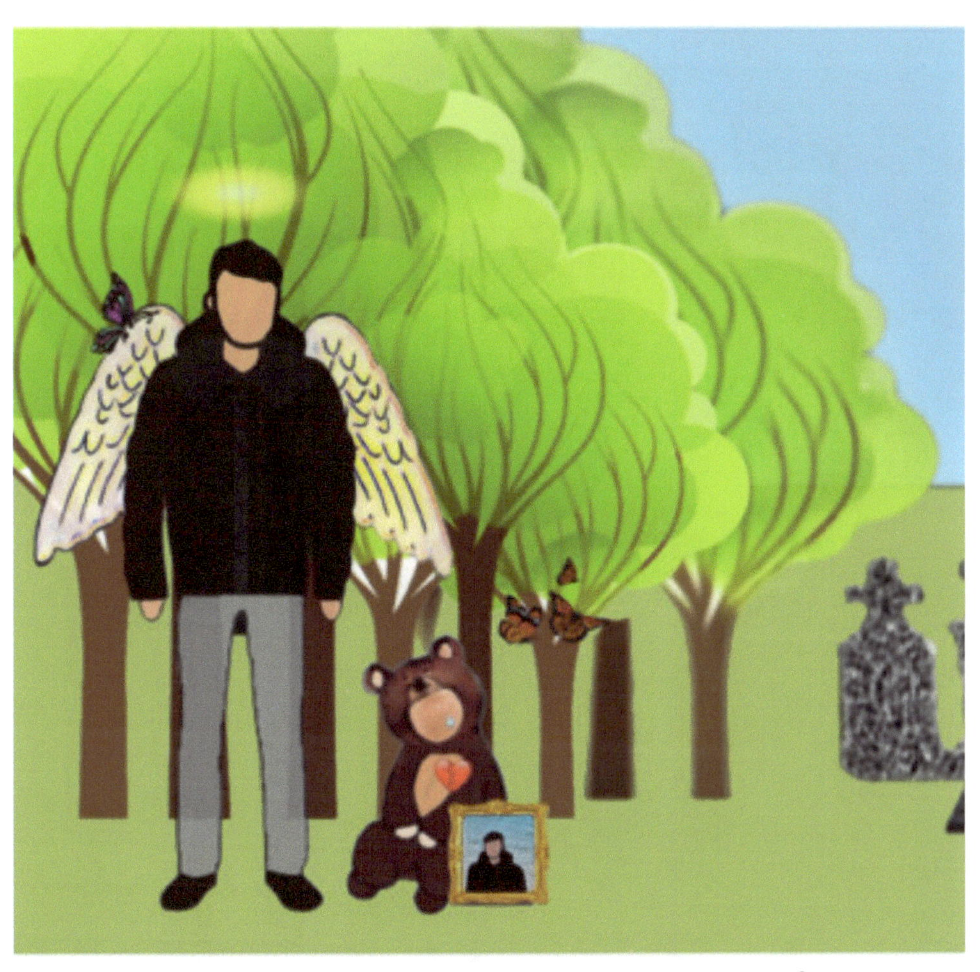

You are in my heart.
And you are all
around.

I wish you were here and
not sleeping in the ground.

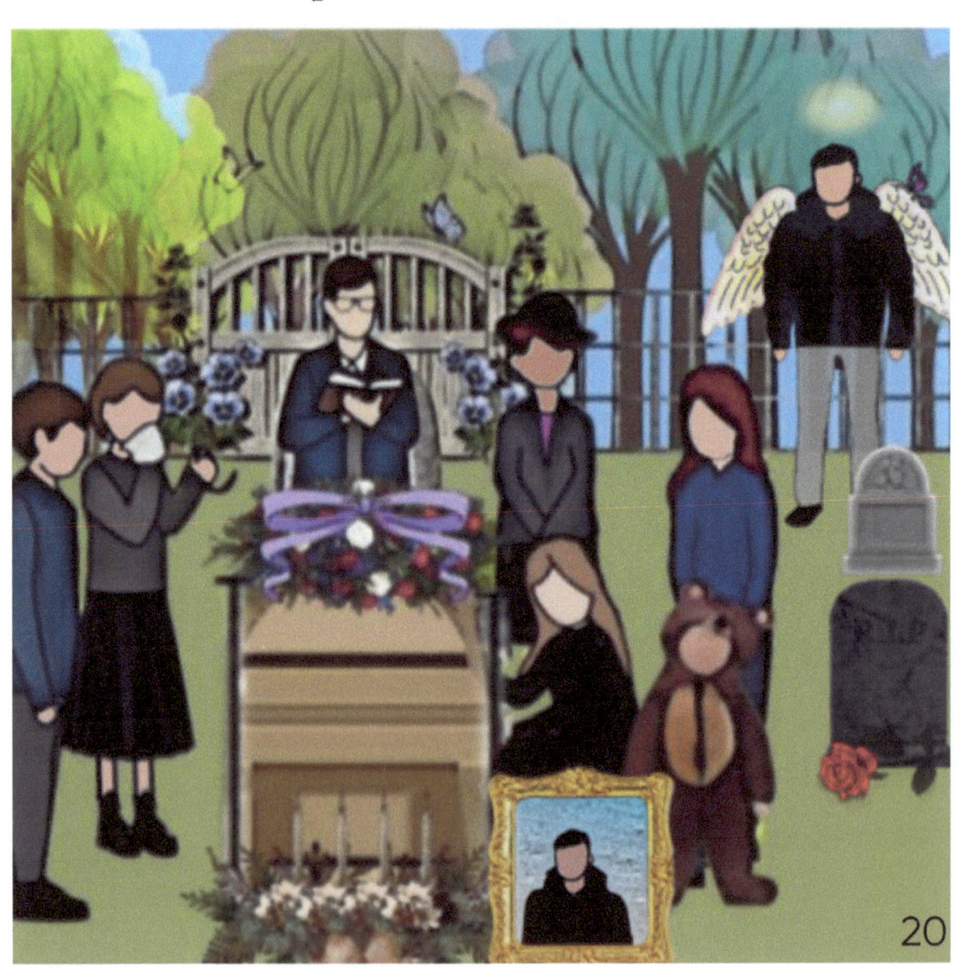

20

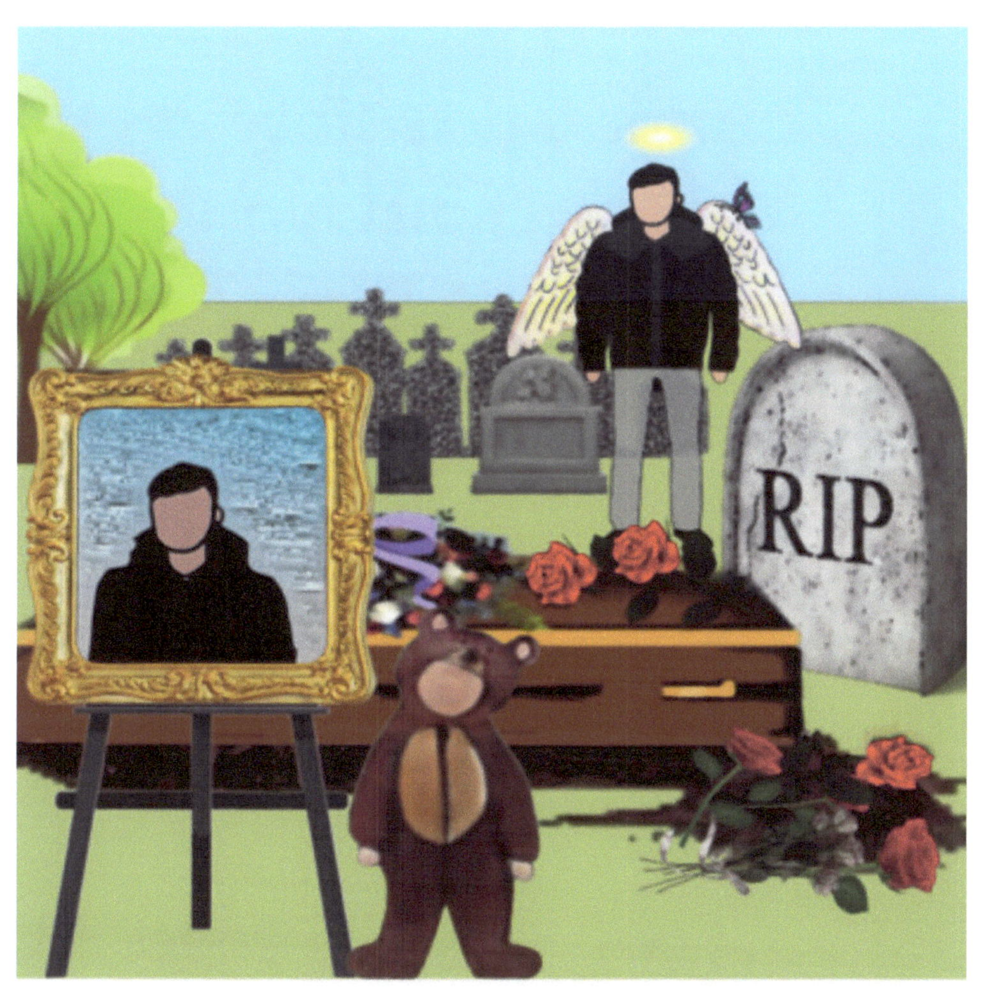

Why are you sleeping?
You had so much do.

I cannot possibly do
this without you.

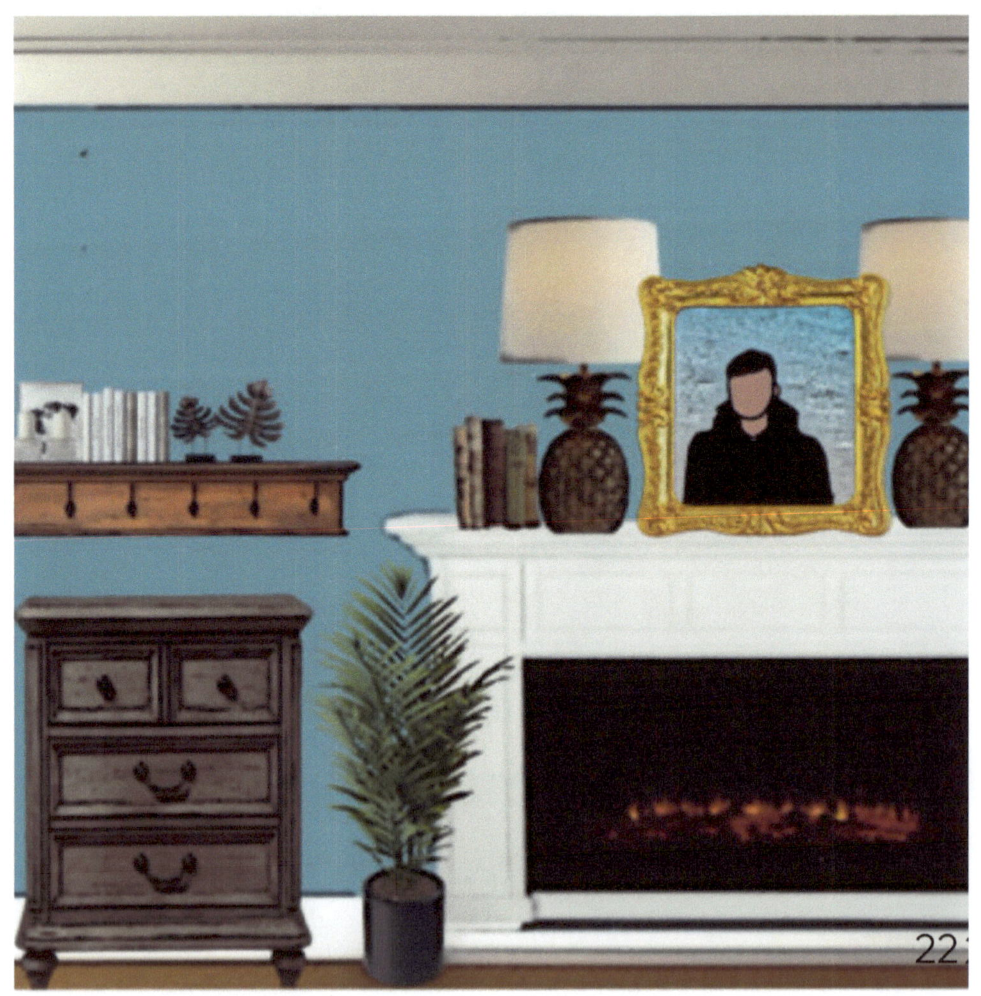

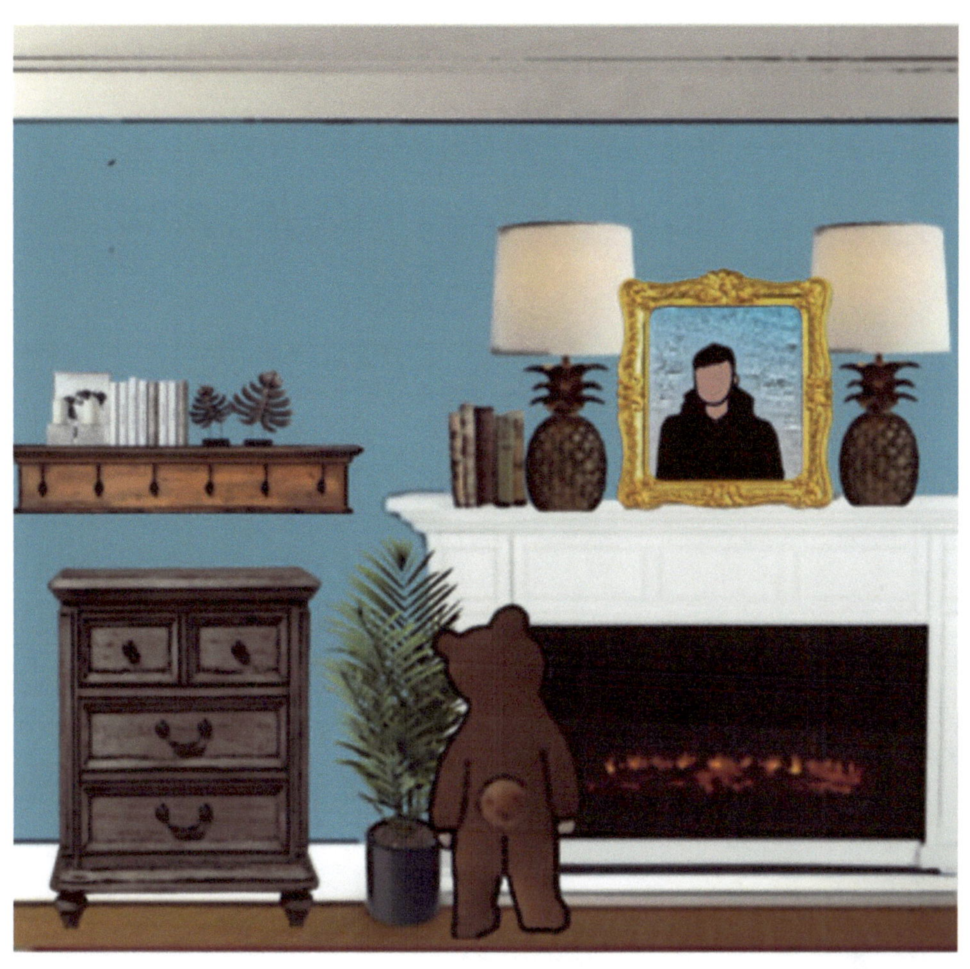

How can I get through life
knowing you're gone?

You're missing milestons
that would have made you
so proud.

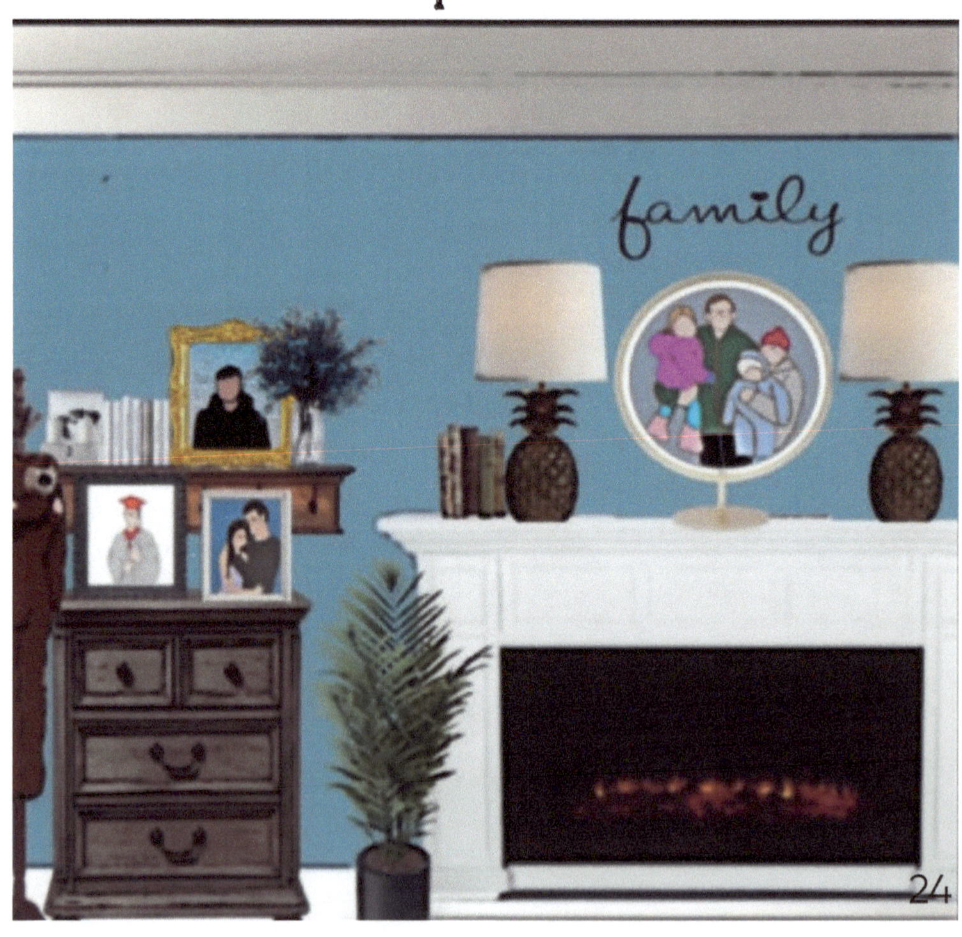

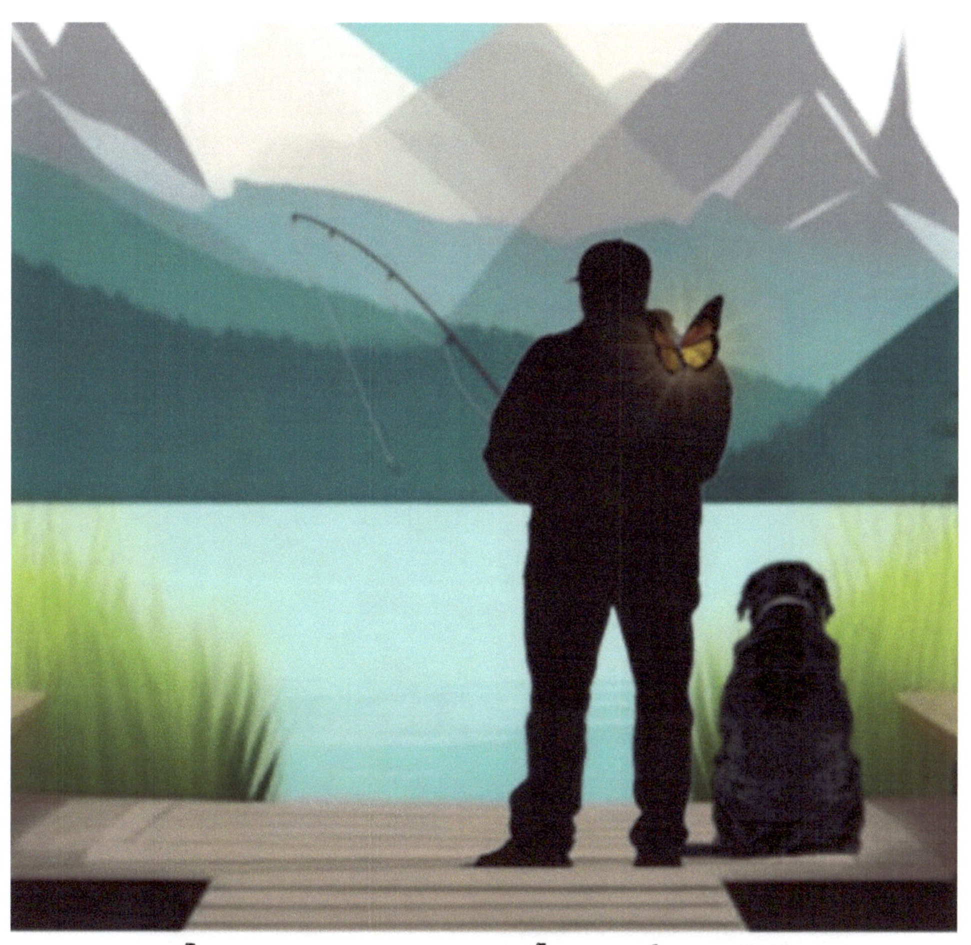

Why are you sleeping? I
know you're still here. I can
feel you in the air, I can
feel you on my skin.

Why are you sleeping? We
were trying to grow. I
know we are family, I
know you're in tow.

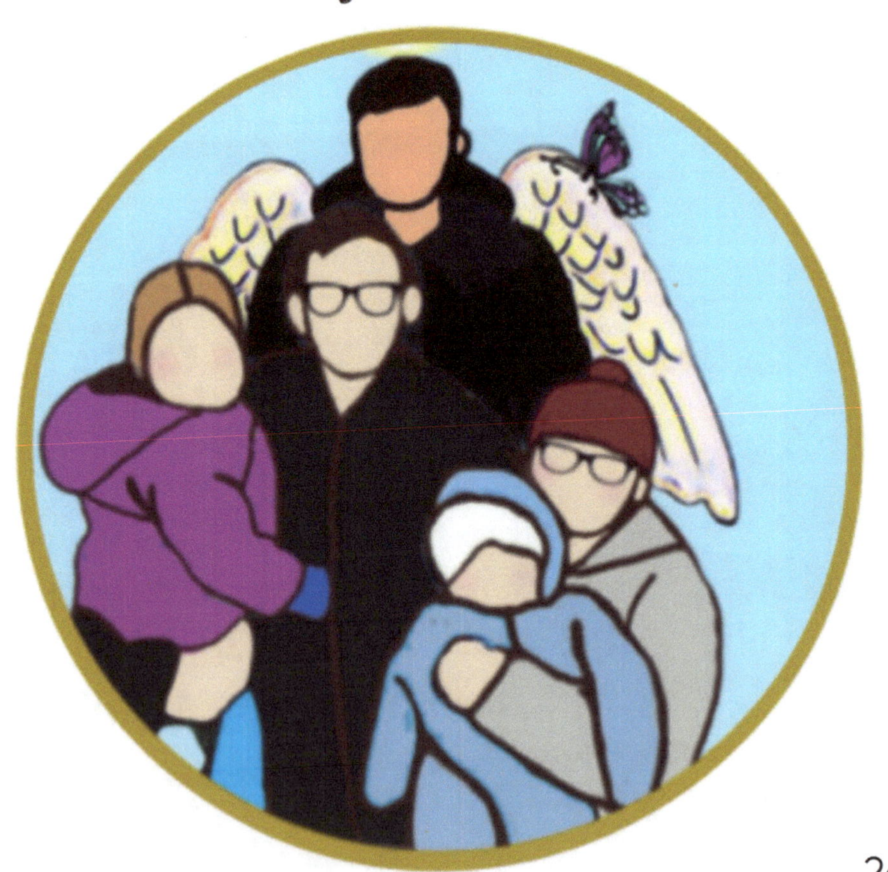

Thank you for being our rock
and our glue.

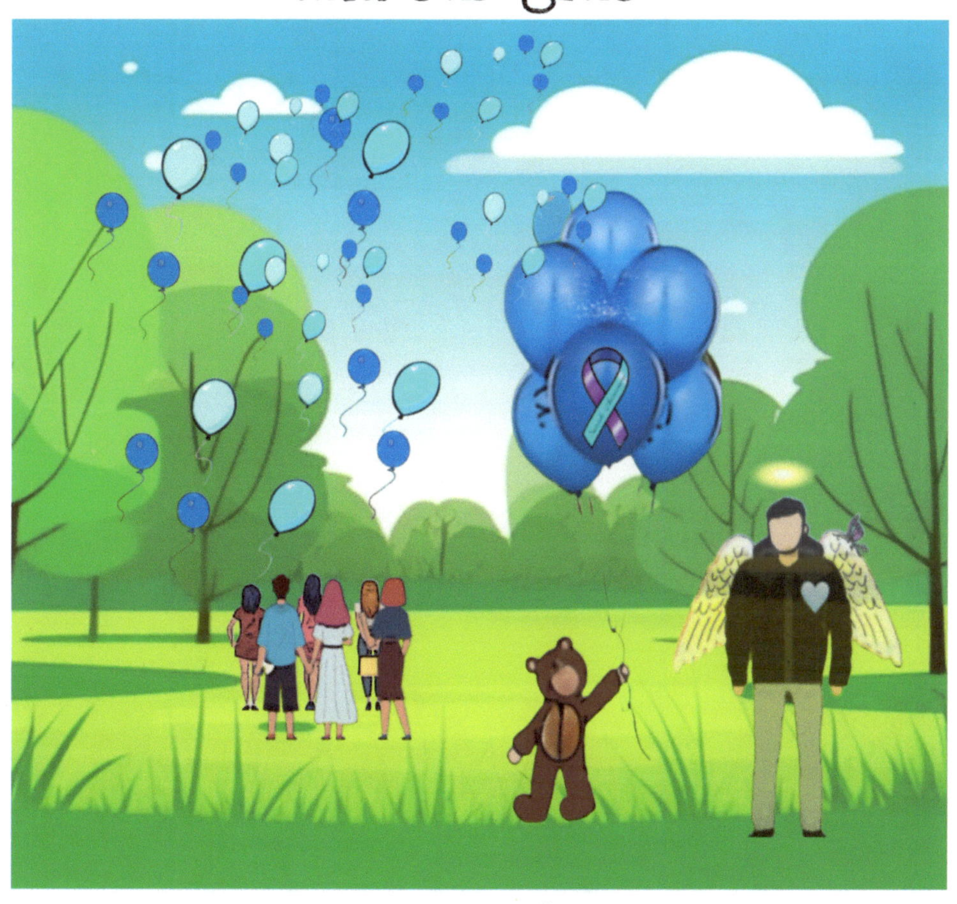

I promise we love you,
through and through!